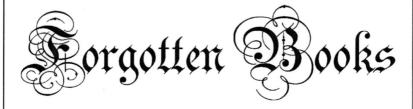
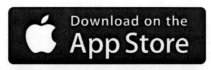
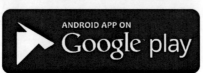

ISBN 978-0-260-19521-0
PIBN 11016502

1 MONTH OF
FREE
READING

at

www.ForgottenBooks.com

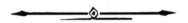

By purchasing this book you are eligible for one month membership to ForgottenBooks.com, giving you unlimited access to our entire collection of over 700,000 titles via our web site and mobile apps.

To claim your free month visit:

www.forgottenbooks.com/free1016502

English
Français
Deutsche
Italiano
Español
Português

www.forgottenbooks.com

Mythology Photography **Fiction**
Fishing Christianity **Art** Cooking
Essays Buddhism Freemasonry
Medicine **Biology** Music **Ancient
Egypt** Evolution Carpentry Physics
Dance Geology **Mathematics** Fitness
Shakespeare **Folklore** Yoga Marketing
Confidence Immortality Biographies
Poetry **Psychology** Witchcraft
Electronics Chemistry History **Law**
Accounting **Philosophy** Anthropology
Alchemy Drama Quantum Mechanics
Atheism Sexual Health **Ancient History**
Entrepreneurship Languages Sport
Paleontology Needlework Islam
Metaphysics Investment Archaeology
Parenting Statistics Criminology
Motivational

Scovill's
Compound Syrup of Sarsaparilla and Stillingia,
OR,
BLOOD AND LIVER SYRUP.

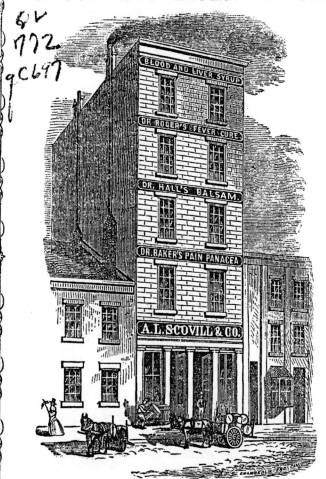

BLOOD AND LIVER SYRUP

DR. ROGER'S FEVER CURE

DR. HALL'S BALSAM.

DR. BAKER'S PAIN PANACEA

A. L. SCOVILL & CO.

FOR THE CURE OF

SCROFULA and all Diseases of the BLOOD and LIVER.

FOR SALE BY

A. L. SCOVILL & CO.,
No. 12 West Eighth Street, Cincinnati, Ohio.

ALSO, WHOLESALE AGENTS FOR

**Dr. Baker's Pain Panacea; Dr. Rogers's Fever Cure; Dr. Mott's
Liver Pills, and Dr. Hall's Balsam.**

SCOVILL'S

COMPOUND EXTRACT OF SARSAPARILLA AND STILLINGIA; OR,

Blood and Liver Syrup,

FOR THE CURE OF

Scrofula, White Swelling, King's Evil, Ulcers, Goitre or Bronchocele, or Swelled Neck, Scrofulous, Diseases, and Indolent Tumors, Mercurial and Syphilitic Affections, Ulcerations and Enlargements of Joints, Glands, Bones or Ovaries, Uterus, Liver, Spleen, Dyspepsia, Liver Complaints, Epileptic Fits, Chorea or St. Vitus's Dance, Dropsy, and all Diseases of the Skin, such as Pimples, Biles, Tetter, or Saltrheum, Ringworm, Sore Eyes; also many diseases peculiar to Females, such as Leucorrhea or Whites, Suppression, Irregularity, Sterility.

THERE is no doubt but there can be found in this climate, Plants containing Medical qualities for ALL the diseases of the country.

But we must first ascertain what their medical action is, both separately and in combination with each other, on the system. They should be procured at times when the Plants contain the greatest amount of active medicinal strength. The *active properties of many plants exist in Salts and Resins, and* CAN NOT BE EXTRACTED BY WATER. I use an Alcoholic Process for extracting the medical qualities.

Read the following statement of WM. S. MERRILL, *the oldest Chemist and Druggist of Cincinnati.*

We hereby certify that we have been made acquainted with the formula of Scovill's Comp. Syrup of **Sarsaparilla and Stillingia**, and it has been made under our supervision. The ingredients are entirely of vegetable origin, and of prime quality, and the virtues extracted in a great measure by an Alcoholic Process. *No mineral substance enters into the composition!*

W. S. MERRILL & CO.,
One door west Burnet House.

It will be seen that the method named for extracting the medicinal virtues of the several agents, viz.: by an ALCOHOLIC PROCESS, etc., is in accordance with the views of our BEST CHEMISTS and PHARMACEUTISTS. *These have, by repeated experiments, established the fact, that with all those medicinal roots containing resinous active constituents, alcohol must be used to obtain them freed from starch, lignin, and other inert matters—water will not answer. Again, they have shown that many roots, barks, etc., which yield* THEIR ACTIVE PRINCIPLES *to water, have these principles dissipated or completely* DESTROYED *by being in contact with heated water for any considerable length of time.* Hence the difficulty in procuring an efficient alterative when prepared by physicians or patients who are not provided with the proper apparatus and means for extracting active principles only ; the efficacy of Sarsaparilla is *greatly impaired by the long boiling to which it is generally subjected,* while the *medicinal virtues of their roots are lost on account of their insolubility in water.* To corroborate my assertions on these points, I would refer to the statements of J. Hancock, M. D., *Philadelphia Journal of Pharmacy, Vol. I, page* 295; of M. Beral, *same Journal, Vol. XV, page* 675; of M. Souberain, *same Journal, Vol. XVI, page* 38, of J. J. Husband, *American Journal of Pharmacy, Vol. XVI, page* 6, etc.

One of the compounds is the addition of **Stillingia**, which is something new in **Sarsaparilla** Compounds, adds GREATLY to its ALTERATIVE VIRTUES, *rendering it thereby much more efficient in eradicating disease.* This plant, although employed by the profession for only a few years, has already attained an *unrivaled reputation as an alterative;* it is a Southern Plant, growing from Virginia to Florida, and was introduced to the profession by THOMAS YOUNG SIMONS, M. D. I would refer those unacquainted with its properties to the statements of the following physicians, all of high standing and extensively known, and who laud it as an *alterative of unequaled efficacy,* viz.: Thomas Y. Simons, M. D., *American Medical Recorder, Vol. XIII, page.* 312 ; A. Lopez, M. D., *New Orleans Medical and Surgical Journal, Vol. III, page* 40 ; and H. R. Frost, M. D., *Southern Journal of Medicine and Pharmacy, Nov.,* 1845. These gentlemen report Stillingia to be *undoubtedly a most valuable remedy in* Scrofula, Cutaneous *Diseases, Secondary Syphilis, Chronic Hepatic Affections,* as well as in many other complaints ordinarily benefited by the use of mercury, and their statements are corroborated by *all physicians* who have tested it.

SCOVILL'S
BLOOD AND LIVER SYRUP!

THIS Medicine is composed of roots and plants which have not only ALTERATIVE, but *Diuretic* and *Diaphoretic Action.* Thus the combination *acts not only on the Blood, but also on the Skin and Kidneys.* It is on this account that my medicine produces so much more speedy action in

ALL CHRONIC DISEASES OF THE SYSTEM,

than any other now before the public. It is an absolute fact, that an Alterative, combined with a Diuretic and Diaphoretic medicine, *will cure many diseases* of a Chronic nature which an Alterative, alone, will not cure ; and, in all cases, *it adds greatly to the action and efficacy of a medicine merely Alterative.*

Is it not reasonable to suppose that, when any part of the system is diseased, and has a *depraved or morbid action,* a medicine which will act on the *Blood,* and also on the secretions of the *Skin* and *Kidneys,* will have a *happier effect* than a medicine acting on the Blood alone. In all *Chronic cases this medicine has almost a specific action.* In fact, it is the only medicine that will *effect a speedy cure* when the system is in a *depraved state.*

IT ACTS ON ALL THE SECRETIONS OF THE SYSTEM,

and, at the same time, *carries off the diseases not only through the Blood, but also through the secretions of the Skin and Kidneys.*

This preparation is compounded upon scientific principles, and with great care, by one thoroughly acquainted with the medical qualities and effects of each article, separately considered, as well as the whole in its combined state. I, therefore, recommend this preparation with the greatest confidence, being fully persuaded that it will give *very general, if not*

UNIVERSAL SATISFACTION.

I do not pretend that it is a *Cure-all,* nor that, in all cases, and under all circumstances, it is absolutely infallible. Common sense teaches us that the *day of miracle has passed,* but *science* and *facts* remain, and on the strength of these we call attention to our

VALUABLE MEDICINE.

The noble science of medicine is controlled by the same powers which govern the entire world. Were my invalid patients simply to take this medicine for a short time, in cases of

Goitre, Cancerous, Scirrhous, or Scrofulous Tumors, Ulceration of the Bones, etc.,

and then drop it, they would receive from it but very little good. They had better not commence its use at all ; for, unless persevered in, the money expended for it is thrown away, nobody is benefited, the disease remains uncured, and the reputation of the medicine is injured. Is it not reasonable to suppose that when the system has been long under the influence of a *Chronic disease,* it would take several months to

ERADICATE IT ENTIRELY FROM THE SYSTEM!

It is necessary to give an explanation of the action of this medicine on the system, which is *through the secretion of the absorbent vessels,* and consists in *receiving or taking up certain substances known as virus,* or *poisonous* principles, and removing them from the diseased parts through the *secretions* and *exhalant arteries,* until they are carried from the system. At the same time *good blood is transported* through the *chyle* to the diseased parts of the body, until the

Entire System is in a Healthy Condition.

The above seems necessary—it being a popular error that a medicine which acts on the Blood must necessarily act also as a Cathartic.

DIRECTIONS FOR USING.

FOR AN ADULT—One tablespoonful three times a day, soon after eating.

FOR A CHILD 10 YEARS OLD—Two large teaspoonfuls three times a day.

FOR A CHILD 4 YEARS OLD—One teaspoonful three times a day.

FOR A CHILD 3 MONTHS OLD—One half-teaspoonful three times a day.

FOR A CHILD 1 MONTH OLD—Twenty drops three times a day.

To be taken in about a wineglassful of sweetened water, if desired.

SOME CONSTITUTIONS REQUIRE EVEN MORE THAN IS NAMED ABOVE, AND SOME LESS. IN ALL CASES, IT SHOULD BE ADMINISTERED UNTIL RESISTED BY THE STOMACH.

SCROFULA OR KING'S EVIL.

This is a morbid state of the LYMPHATIC GLANDULAR SYSTEM. At first small knots appear under the skin, behind the ears, or on the neck, which gradually increase in size and number, until they run together into one large hard TUMOR. This often continues for a long time without breaking, and even then it only discharges a thin watery humor. Sometimes these knots appear on the GROINS ARMPITS, FEET, HANDS, EYES, BREASTS, LIPS, AND NOSE. TREATMENT.—Take a dose of this medicine three times a day—morning, noon, and night—about one-half hour after eating, and gradually increase them if the stomach will permit. In case there is a TUMOR or SWELLING, a cure may be facilitated by using an OINTMENT, which can be procured at a Druggist's, composed as follows : Iodide of Potassium 3ss., Lard 3iss. Dissolve the Iodide of Potassium in 3 or 4 drops of water (or more if necessary.) After being finely powdered, mix it thoroughly with the Lard. At first use one half drachm twice a day, or a piece the size of half a nutmeg. With this rub the parts affected. If they become tender, it may be omitted for a day or two; but continue taking the medicine until the cure is effected. A nutritious diet should be used, and out-door exercise if the patient can bear it. Should there be SCROFULOUS ULCERS, with pain, get the IODINE OINTMENT made as follows :

R Iodine, xv grains.   Morphine, v grains.
   Iodide of Potassium, 3i.   Lard, 3 ii.

Powder the Iodine and Iodide of Potassium fine and dissolve in 5 or 6 drops of water (or more if necessary); then mix thoroughly with the Lard, to be applied to the parts affected. Spread it on thin cloth, and change every day.

CANCER.

This disease is known by the blue veins like crab's claws. It usually attacks glandular portions of the body, such as the BREAST, NOSE, EYES, NECK, and TONGUE.

SYMPTOMS.—It is first attended by a peculiar burning, shooting, or darting pain, and discoloration of the skin.

TREATMENT.—Give a dose of this medicine three times a day, and apply the following Ointment:

R Iodide of Potassium, 3ss.   Morphine, v grains,   Cerate, 3 i.

Powder the Iodide of Potassium, dissolve in 8 drops of water, and then mix with the Morphine and Lard. Spread thin on a piece of linen and apply to the parts affected. If they are inflamed, apply a poultice of Flaxseed, Slippery Elm, or Bread and Milk, instead of the Ointment, until the inflammation is out. Afterward, apply the Ointment again.

BRONCHOCELE, OR GOITRE (SWELLED NECK).

SYMPTOMS.—It is known by the enlargement of the THYROID GLAND. This gland lies over or near the front of the neck and each side of the windpipe, just below the middle of the neck. GOITRE is often larger than persons, not familiar with the disease, would suppose them to be from their external appearance, as they are bound down by the muscles on each side of the neck.

R Iodide of Potassium, 3ss.   Lard, 3 i.

Powder the Iodide of Potassium finely, then dissolve in 8 drops of water, and mix thoroughly with the Lard. Take at first about the size of half a nutmeg and rub into the TUMOR, and gradually increase to double that amount each day. Continue to take the medicine and use the Ointment until a cure is effected.

WENS to be treated the same as we have treated GOITRE.

MERCURIAL AND SYPHILITIC DISEASES.

SYMPTOMS.—Its attack is mostly on the THROAT, MOUTH, and NOSE · *but no part of the body is exempt from its ravages,*

TREATMENT —Take a dose of this medicine three times a day, and continue until you are entirely cured. This medicine is ABSORBED by the FLUIDS into the BLOOD VESSELS, and changes the *morbid poisons to a healthy condition of the blood, until the diseases are entirely eradicated from the system.*

IN ULCERATION OF THE THROAT OR MOUTH it will greatly facilitate the cure to gargle the mouth or throat with No. 6, or which is much better, *Dr. Baker's Pain Panacea* mixed with a little water.

WHITE SWELLINGS,

OR SCROFULOUS AND RHEUMATIC ULCERATION OF THE JOINTS.

SYMPTOMS.—This disease originates in the SYNOVIAL MEMBRANE, which often arises from cold. This disease is known by such TUMORS as primarily AFFECT THE BONES, and then the LIGAMENTS and SOFT JOINTS. And in other cases the CARTILAGES, LIGAMENT and soft parts become diseased before there is any *morbid affection* of the BONES.

TREATMENT.—Take a dose of this medicine three times a day, at the same time dress the part affected with IODINE OINTMENT, as we recommend in *Scrofulous Ulcers.* After worn a week, it may be changed to one made of STRAMONIUM OINTMENT, which can be had at any Druggist's, or may be made by taking a handful of green leaves and stewing them in fresh lard, and then strained. This may be worn a week, and then change again for the Iodine Ointment, and so alternatively. After using this medicine a few months, and the sores commence to heal, you may make the following HEALING OINTMENT :

℞ Linseed Oil, One Pint,   Spirits Turpentine, two tablespoonfuls,
Red Lead, ℥ii,   Strained Honey, two tablespoonfuls.
Beeswax, ℥ii.

Put the oil and red lead into an iron vessel and boil slowly until it commences to smoke ; then pour off and dissolve the beeswax in it. When it commences to cool, add the honey and spirits of turpentine. Spread on thin cloth, and apply to the ulcers. Wash the parts every other day with Castile soap and water.

This HEALING OINTMENT is the MOST VALUABLE one for *healing* that has ever been discovered. Any OLD SORES that have baffled ALL OTHER TREATMENT will yield to this.

EPILEPSY, AND CONVULSIONS OR FITS.

In young persons this disease may be cured by this medicine. And many adults are greatly benefited so long as they continue to use it. Dose, three times a day.

ERYSIPELAS, OR ST. ANTONY'S FIRE.

In acute form, make a cranberry poultice, and apply to the parts. This will generally relieve in a short time. In CHRONIC form, take this medicine three a day. In most cases, if persevered in, *it will cure.*

TETTER, OR SALTRHEUM,

Take this medicine three times a day, and use an Ointment made of the following :
Take Iodide Potassium, ℥i,
" Lard, ℥i.

Make as directed under the head Scrofula, or King's Evil, and apply to the parts affected, twice a day.

LIVER COMPLAINT.

SYMPTOMS.—In acute form, there is pain in the side, just under the lower rib, frequently of a dull or obtuse character; sometimes there is pain over the shoulders; sometimes, when lying on the left side, there is a general uneasiness, attended with a difficulty of breathing. CHRONIC FORM is characterized by an *unhealthy complexion, loss of appetite and flesh, Costiveness, Indigestion, Flatulence (belching of wind from the stomach), Pain in the Stomach, a Yellowness of the Eyes and Skin* ; also an obtuse pain in the region of the liver, extending to the shoulder. In many cases, on post mortem examination, it has been found they had come to their death, from an *abscess of the liver,* although they had suffered no great inconvenience while living.

TREATMENT.—Take a dose of this medicine three times a day ; at the same time rub freely over the region of the liver once or twice a day with salt mixed with alcohol. Care should be used as to the diet. Eat nothing but what agrees with the stomach. Also regular exercise should be taken in the open air, between meals. The bowels should be kept open. If necessary, use DR. MOTT'S VEGETABLE LIVER PILLS, which will be found a valuable assistant.

DYSPEPSIA, OR INDIGESTION.

This disease is generally brought on by overloading the stomach, eating just before going to bed, sedentary habits, or want of proper exercise. It may be a long time coming on, without seeming to exist.

SYMPTOMS.—A distress in the stomach after *eating, nausea, heartburn, flatulency, loss of appetite, a gnawing in the stomach when empty, a pain in the side or breast,* great *costiveness, paleness of the countenance, languor,* an *unwillingness* to move about, *low spirits, palpitations,* and *disturbed sleep.*

TREATMENT.—Take a dose of this medicine three times a day, and rub briskly over the liver and stomach once a day with salt mixed with alcohol. Great pains should in all cases be observed as to the diet. The stomach should never be overloaded. No meal should ever be finished. Always leave off eating before the appetite is appeased. Never eat before going to bed. Take free exercise in the open air. If the stomach is sour, take (Dr. Physic's Ley) as follows : *Wood soot, six ounces ; pure wood ashes, one quart; and mix one gallon of boiling water.* Let it stand twelve hours, then pour off and bottle; Take one tablespoonful after each meal. If you are costive, your bowels should be kept open by using DR. MOTT'S VEGETABLE LIVER PILLS, by taking one or more every night.

SCROFULOUS CONSUMPTION.

TREATMENT.—Take a dose of this medicine three times a day. If this should not raise the phlegm easy, you can make an expectorant, as follows :

R *Hive Syrup, Зi,* *Syrup of Squills, Зi,*
  Tinct, Blood Root, Зii, *Acetate Morphine, grains ii.*

Mix, and take one teaspoonful every hour until it produces a free expectoration. After this is produced, take the expectorate three times a day, and continue the medicine.

DROPSY.

Take a dose of this medicine three times a day. At the same time take the following : One half a pound of squills in two quarts of good cider. Let it stand six days, and after that time take one tablespoonful twice a day. This, with the medicine, will excite the flow of the urine, by acting on the absorbient vessels, and carrying the fluid away.

RHEUMATISM.

In Acute Rheumatism you can get the following STIMULATING LINIMENT put up by some Druggist :

R *Oil Origanum,* *Strong Spirits Camphor,*
  " *Hemlock,* " " *Ammonia,*
  " *Sassafras,* *Laudanum—each Зss.*

Mix this together. Bathe the parts affected by rubbing it in twice a day briskly with a piece of flannel for fifteen minutes. When the pain is severe, heat a shovel and hold it over the parts while bathing ; and if the pain continues long, take this medicine three times a day.

CHRONIC RHEUMATISM.—Use this stimulating liniment twice a day, and take this medicine three times a day. If you cannot procure the stimulating liniment, get Dr. Baker's Pain Panacea, which will answer a good purpose in its place.

NEURALGIA AND GOUT.—To be treated the same as Rheumatism.

PARALYSIS, OR PALSY.

Use the STIMULATING LINIMENT, (as directed in RHEUMATISM) and take a dose three times a day of this medicine.

SUPPRESSED MENSES,

By neglecting to attend to this disease, young persons are brought in thousands a premature grave. Take DR. MOTT'S VEGETABLE LIVER PILLS sufficient to operate on the bowels freely every night about the expected time, and on going to bed soak the feet in warm water and *drink freely* of *Pennyroyal Tea;* also, take a dose of this medicine twice a day. As much out-door exercise should be taken as the system will bear. If this treatment is persevered in, a cure is certain.

SCALD HEAD.

Take a little Stramonium Ointment—(The directions for making this can be found under the head of White Swelling, or it may be had of some Druggist)—and anoint the parts affected every other day. Wash the parts also once each week with warm water and Castile soap, and take a dose of this medicine twice a day. This treatment is a specific, and was never known to fail.

ULCERS, OR OLD SORES,

Of all kinds, use this medicine three times a day. If the ulcers are inflamed, make a poultice of slippery elm, flaxseed, or bread and milk, and when the inflammation is out you may use the Healing Ointment, (see under head of White Swelling,) and in exchange use the Stramonium Ointment (see under the head of White Swellings.) If this course is persevered in, a cure is certain.

SYPHILITIC, AND SWELLING OF THE BONES.

Use this medicine three times a day, and at the same time use the following ointment.

Take Iodine, ℈ii,   Take Emp. Soap, ℥ii.
" Iodine Potassium, ℈ss,

Mix, and apply to the parts affected by spreading the Ointment on thin cloth.

BOILS.

Take a dose of this medicine three times a day; and if the system is weak, take one teaspoonful of carb. iron, mixed with a little water, twice a day.

CHLOROSIS, OR OBSTRUCTIONS IN FEMALES.

Take a dose of this medicine three times a day; and also use one or more of DR. MOTT'S VEGETABLE LIVER PILLS every night, just sufficient to keep the bowels regular.

ENLARGEMENT OF THE HEART AND LIVER.

Take a dose of this medicine three times a day. All stimulating drinks should be avoided.

ENLARGEMENT OF THE BONES AND JOINTS.

Take a dose of this medicine three times a day, and use the Stimulating Liniment as directed for Rheumatism. If the disease should not yield, use the IODINE PAINT twice a week.

IODINE PAINT.

R Take Iodine, ℥i.   Iodide of Potassium, ℈ss.   Alcohol, ℥i.
Paint the parts effectually with a common hair pencil.

JAUNDICE.

Take this medicine three times a day, and drink at the same time one tumbler of sour cider, and take two drops of Oil of Juniper every night. Rub briskly over the Liver with salt and alcohol before going to bed.

LEUCORRHEA, OR WHITES.

This disease attacks females of all ages. TREATMENT.—Use this medicine three times a day, and use DR. MOTT'S LIVER PILLS every other night. Use an injection made of Oak Bark, or take one ounce of Nutgalls (bruised) and steep in one pint of hot water, and use 4 or 6 Female-Syringefulls at night.

DISEASE OF THE SKIN.

Take this medicine three times a day, and, if there is much itching of the skin, use at night, on the parts affected, the *Ointment of Iod. Potassium*, until the itching is relieved.

DISEASE OF THE KIDNEYS.

Take this medicine three times a day, and bathe freely over the parts with salt and alcohol on going to bed.

THE FOLLOWING EXPLANATION SHOWS HOW SCOVILL'S
BLOOD AND LIVER SYRUP
Cures Diseases, by carrying out of the Blood, through the Secretions, all Impurities.

· PLATE 1.

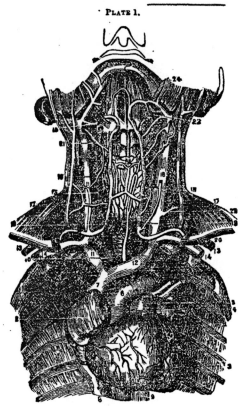

EXPLANATION TO PLATE 1.

This cut illustrates a view of the **heart and the great blood-vessels** which play such an important part in the constitution and action of the system. All the material which is taken into the system, from which healthy matter, either for removal of disease or for the natural support of the system, is taken up by the absorbents which are so abundantly spread over the parts of the body, as seen also in plates 2, 3, 5, and conveyed into the general circulation. The stomach, like the parts illustrated, being thus provided with the same absorbents, it is important, in curing diseases, to use such medicines as will agree with the stomach, so as to be taken up also by the absorbents, that the **general circulation of the blood may be improved** and changed by the admission of healthy material, which cures disease, by being admitted into the blood. Now, if poisons be given, the stomach rejects them to a certain extent; and even the small portion which is taken into the blood produces a very dangerous condition, and often remains so firmly fixed in the system, that it requires months to remove it; and, in fact, in some cases it is almost impossible to remove it altogether. This is the case with all the mercurial preparations, one of which, in most common use, is calomel. If this or any other poison enter the system in this way, to cure or remove them, medicine of a healthy character must be used in the same way. Our medicine fulfills this want without fail. It not only acts so as **to carry the diseased matter from the blood,** but keeps the heart itself in a healthy condition.

In every part of the system there are three continuous actions going on—circulation, nutrition, and secretion. These three actions are co1 mon to every system, and are regular and uniform in their results. We mean, by the **circulation,** a fluid denominated blood-lymph or sap, deposited in the various tissues, and subsequently retaken from them, of the materials of which all the fluids and solids of the body are formed. These solids and fluids become blended together; in this way **the blood becomes organized, and endowed with life and vitality.**

The **nutrition** is an action in the several parts of the solids of the body, receiving from and returning to the parts the particles of matter which are necessary to keep the body in a condition equal to the state before the natural changes take place; in other words, it **prevents the body from decreasing or wasting away;** this action supplies from the blood material which sustains and keeps up the health of the parts, equal to that which is carried out of the system as matter unfit longer to remain. As all the materials for nourishing the system, or keeping the body in health, are derived from the blood, it is impossible, **if the blood is diseased, to have a healthy body. The** life of each part is involved in the **life** of the whole body; and in order that the life of the blood, as well as the life of other parts constituting the life of the body may be preserved, every change must be **watched** with great care. Any departure from the above rule, will result in disease. If the natural supply of blood received by any part of the body be altered in any respect, it will cause a change in that part. **If the blood is impure,** in any respect, parts of the body will be diseased in proportion to the extent of **the change.** Healthy blood will excite the brain,

PLATE 2.

PLATE 3.

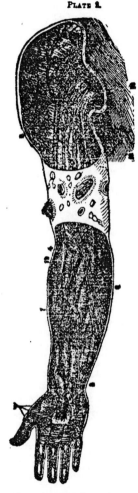

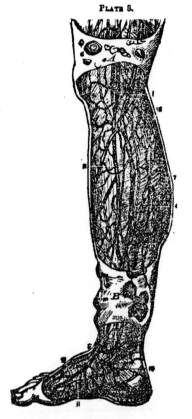

EXPLANATION TO PLATE 2.

Plate 2 represents the arm, with **its blood - vessels and absorbents.** There is also a portion of the flesh and skin, illustrating a diseased condition. From this it will be seen that the direct supply the skin receives is from the blood-vessels as well as from the absorbents. Now, if the blood is diseased, the skin can not be cured. All the local applications of medicine that could be made will not cure skin diseases, unless medicine is used to purify the blood and supply the skin with **a sufficient amount of healthy blood.** Hence the necessity of using medicines which will cure **all** skin diseases in this way.

EXPLANATION TO PLATE 3.

This cut illustrates fully the leg, the blood-vessels, lymphatics, and all the deep-seated vessels. Letter B **represents an ulcer, which is nothing but a diseased condition of the part,** wherever located. Now, this may extend to the flesh only, or it may extend to the bone also, and produce the condition found in **Martin Robbins's case.** (See his certificate on one of the following pages.) The letter A, in this plate, illustrates a diseased condition of the skin similar to that in the arm of plate 2. To cure them, the blood must be made healthy. Nothing can be more clear to our minds, from a careful examination of the body, anatomically and physiologically, than that we have now adopted the only true theory of curing chronic diseases. **Our medicines** are prepared in view of a perfect knowledge of the facts in the case.

as the great center and life of the nervous system, to perform all its natural action. By this the lungs are made to act, breathing is regular and easy, and the heart and pulse act regularly. This keeps the blood circulating equally in all parts of the body ; and keeping the body in a natural warmth, the stomach digests the food, the liver secretes the bile, the bowels act as they should, the kidneys perform their duty by throwing off the urine, see fig. 6, Plate 4.

While this is going on, every thing is thrown from the body which will not make the parts healthy, or give it strength. Now, if the blood be diseased, the brain will not be stimulated to act ; then the lungs, stomach, liver, bowels, and kidneys are all impaired in their action, the result of which is, that some of the most dangerous diseases are firmly seated.

PLATE 4.

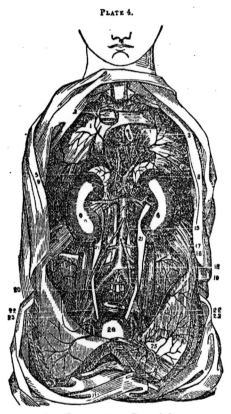

EXPLANATION TO PLATE 4.

This illustrates the kidneys and the large blood-vessels connected with them. Figure 6 is the kidneys. These are secreting organs, and have to carry from the blood morbid or diseased material, which must be taken from the system. If, in a healthy man, the secretion, which should be carried off by the kidneys, be stopped for seventy hours, the man would die by the accumulation of the uric acid, which is poisonous, if retained in the blood in large quantity. Now, if the arrest of the action of the kidneys entirely will destroy life in so short a time, we know, if they are injured in their action even to a small degree, the person becomes diseased. Figure 21 represents the small tubes leading from the kidneys to the bladder. It is through these that the urine passes into the bladder after it is formed in the kidney. It is just as important to have the kidneys act in order to cure diseases, as it is for the stomach or heart to act. In our combination of agents to make a Blood and Liver Syrup, we have had special reference to this point ; in this our expectation and intention has been realized, for no medicine is found to work more efficiently, and with more certainty, than this.

When the blood is too poor in quality, or too scarce in quantity, it produces a variety of diseases. When the quantity of blood in the lungs is too great for the quantity of air breathed in a given time, it becomes rapidly diseased. If a person breathes twenty-one or twenty-two times in a minute, as a general rule, the pulse will be about seventy-five. If the pulse increases up to one hundred and twenty or one hundred and forty, and the breathing continues the same, it will be seen, at once, that this will destroy the blood rapidly, as it becomes thin and impure ; the heart continues to force it through the system faster and faster, until the healthy part of it is taken to supply the body until it has become so very poor that the brain, for want of stimulus which the blood alone can give, ceases to act, and the individual dies.

There is no other way to cure diseases but by first purifying the whole system so as to create a healthy circulation.

The first medical men of the age agree with us, that no disease of any extent can be cured without using such medicines as will act directly upon the blood. Why many medical men have failed to cure chronic diseases is, because the medicines used have not been such as will act beneficially on the blood.

The many thousands of bottles which have been used by the public, and the many gallons and barrels supplied to the physicians, warrant us in saying, that during the last two years we have been more successful with our Blood and Liver Syrup in curing hopeless cases of chronic diseases than have any other remedies in the hands of physicians or before the public.

It is now admitted that no other combination known to the profession, acts so promptly upon diseases as our medicine.

Not a single physician, out of many hundreds who have given it a fair trial, so far as we are informed, has abandoned its use; but, on the contrary, they admit all we have claimed for it. One physician informs us that he has used it with entire success during the last few years, in hundreds of cases, such as **Scrofula, Syphilitic and Mercurial Disease, White Swelling, and other Chronic diseases,** many of which were deep-seated, and all other remedies had failed to cure. If the real merits of this remedy could be known, twelve months would not pass until the greater portion of the **thirty-five thousand Physicians** now in the United States would be using it in preference to any other remedy in diseases for which it is recommended.

PLATE 5.

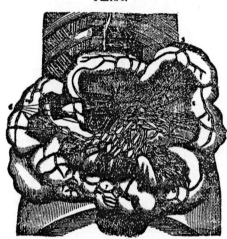

EXPLANATION TO PLATE 5.

Plate 5 shows how abundantly the intestines are supplied with absorbents. In fact, no part is without them. Every medicine taken into the system, that acts in concert with it, acts more or less upon this delicate structure.

We say this from the testimony given in favor of the use of the Blood and Liver Syrup by numbers of medical men who have used it in treating chronic cases.

Our medicine acts in perfect harmony with all the different organs of the body—with the **lungs, stomach, liver, kidney,** and especially as an alterative on the system.

Having placed this medicine before the public, we challenge any and all **medical investigation and science** that may be brought against it. We know its effect upon the human system, in **removing from the blood all the impurities** which result in consequence of diseases.

Our Blood and Liver Syrup is an officinal preparation, approved of by the **very best physicians** from all parts. Even **professors in medical colleges** have adopted it in their hospital cases where other medicines have failed.

SCOVILL'S BLOOD AND LIVER SYRUP

is composed of medical roots and plants which have not only **alterative but diuretic and diaphoretic action.** Thus the combination acts not only on the blood, but also on the **skin and kidneys.** It is on this account that it produces more of **specific action in chronic diseases** than any other remedy now before the public. Is it not reasonable to suppose, that when any part of the system is diseased, and has **depraved and morbid action,** a medicine which will act on the blood, and also on the secretions of the skin and the kidneys, will have a happier effect than a medicine acting on the blood alone? **It carries off the disease not only through the blood, but also through the skin and kidneys.**

This preparation is compounded upon scientific principles, and with great care. We do not pretend that it is a cure-all, nor that, in all cases, and under all circumstances, it is absolutely infallible. Common sense teaches us that **the day of miracles** has passed, but science and facts remain, and on the strength of these we call attention to our **Blood and Liver Syrup.** The noble science of medicine is controlled by the same powers which govern the entire world. Were the invalid patients simply to take this medicine for a short time, in cases of **goitre, syphilitic,** or **scrofulous tumors, ulceration of the bones, etc.,** and then drop it, they would receive from it but very little good; for unless **persevered in,** the money expended for it is comparatively thrown away, nobody is benefited, the disease remains uncured, and the reputation of the medicine is injured. The action of the medicine is through the secretion of the absorbent vessels, which consists in receiving or taking up certain substances **known as virus, or poisonous principles,** and removing them from the diseased parts through the secretions and exhalants, until they are carried from the system; at the same time **good blood is transported** through the vessels to the diseased parts of the body.

Thus it will **most positively** be seen that it is **impossible for disease of the blood to remain in the system** if the use of this medicine is persevered in, except in cases where the disease has worked on the system so much that there is not vitality enough left for recuperation.

READ HIS STATEMENTS!

A WONDERFUL CURE

— OF —

SCROFULOUS WHITE SWELLING!

Read what Dr. R. S. NEWTON says.

" While young Robbins was in the very worst imaginable condition, I called to attend him for a fracture of the leg, produced by a fall. The indications of a reunion of the bone, under the circumstances, were very unfavorable, for he would sit, day after day, *picking out small pieces of the bone which would slough off.* I found him using **SCOVILL'S** preparation, which he continued to use until a cure was effected. We gave him no constitutional treatment, being in attendance only as a surgeon ; yet we confess we had much curiosity to see what could be done in a system so extensively diseased as his was."

When MARTIN ROBBINS *was cured,* so remarkable was the nature of his case, that DR. NEWTON procured some of SCOVILL'S BLOOD AND LIVER SYRUP to use in his private practice in treating chronic cases. Such was the astonishing success, that he came to the conclusion it should be known to the profession, and speaking of the properties of SCOVILL'S BLOOD AND LIVER SYRUP, he voluntarily published the formula and his (M. Robbins') statements, in the *Medical Journal,* May number, 1859, page 310.

MESSRS. A. L. SCOVILL & CO.:   CINCINNATI, FEBRUARY 16, 1858.

Gentlemen : I will, with great pleasure, give my testimony as to what your SARSAPARILLA AND STILLINGIA, or BLOOD AND LIVER SYRUP, has done for me. Some three and a half years since, I was attacked with a **Scrofulous White Swelling,** which was attended with *most excruciating pains.* I tried various remedies, and had *two of the best physicians* of the city, (one of them a Professor in an Old School Medical College,) and they *failed to give me any relief.* I was so reduced that I was confined to my bed for over three months. The nerves and muscles of one leg were so contracted and drawn up that **I could not walk.** I had more than a dozen running ulcers on my legs, from which I took, from time to time, more than one hundred pieces of bone, some of them from three to four inches long. I was reduced to almost a skeleton, and my friends *had given up all hopes of my recovery.* I was in this condition when I commenced the use of your BLOOD AND LIVER SYRUP. I have used, altogether, some two dozen bottles of it, and at the same time the IODINE OINTMENT, which you advise to use with it; and lastly, the HEALING OINTMENT, given under the head of " **White Swelling,** " in your directions. I am now able to attend to business, and my legs have become so strong that I walk without any difficulty, and have entirely recovered my health !
    Yours, truly,   MARTIN ROBBINS, JR.
Residence on Eighth street, between Mound and John, No. 321; or at place of business, with BROWN & VALLETTE, *No. 4 East Fourth Street.*

TESTIMONY OF WELL-KNOWN CITIZENS.

CINCINNATI, *February* 16, 1858.

WE, the undersigned, are acquainted with MR. MARTIN ROBBINS, JR., and his statement is entitled to the *entire confidence* of the public.
        Yours, most respectfully,
     W. S. MERRELL, *Wholesale Druggist, one door west of the Burnet House.*
     C. F. HALL, *Seal Manufactory,* 14 *West Fourth street.*
     J. C. SHROYER, *Drug Grinder, corner of Fifth and Home streets.*

READ THE STATEMENT OF A HIGHLY RESPECTABLE DRUGGIST.

DIRECTED TO

DR. R. S. NEWTON.

SCROFULA OF THE WORST FORM!

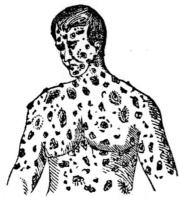

NEW WASHINGTON, CRAWFORD Co., O., Jan. 24. 60.

I send you a statement which is correct. A young man in this place, who had the Scrofula so bad that the doctors gave him up and considered his case incurable, tried all remedies he could hear of. His mother came in my store, and wanted to know if I had anything that would cure him. I recommended Scovill's Blood and Liver Syrup. She took one bottle, and since that has got two more.

The first bottle got him on his feet, and the second enabled him to walk; the third she got this morning.

He was the worst living human being you ever saw. He would frighten the firmest minded man. He was paler than any corpse I ever saw; he had sores on him larger than my fist, in different places. The above is a true statement. His skin has now a good color, and he feels well. He was actually the worst looking living being I ever saw; a man could hardly look at him without shedding tears.

Yours,   W. H. PRATT, D_ruggist.

☞ We cut the following from the *Medical Journal*, a monthly periodical published in Cincinnati. It is from the pen of the editor, **Professor R. S. NEWTON.** This *Journal* is the exponent of one of our prominent **MEDICAL INSTITUTIONS,** and its EDITOR, a prominent **Physician and Professor** in the Institution alluded to, says:

"If the people want a popular medicine, they have one here, composed of the very best agents, made in the most careful manner, after an approved formula. We have known the manufacturers of it personally for many years, and can say that they are reliable men. The formula given is greatly superior to any other alterative now before the public.

"We have used Scovill's Compound Syrup of Sarsaparilla and Stillingia, both private and in the worst kind of Hospital cases, in large quantities, and find it in every instance to accomplish the desired object. This is now one of the officinal medicines. Hundreds of physicians will refuse even the best of medicines, while the combination is unknown, who would willingly adopt its use when made acquainted with the formula for its preparation.

"Messrs. SCOVILL & CO.'S Compound is now as much a regular officinal preparation, as any in the United States Dispensatory, and in this respect they occupy a different position from any other men who are preparing medicine for the public. A highly important point in their preparation of this compound, is their extensive facilities in procuring the several articles during the seasons when they contain the greatest amount of medicinal powers.

"We have examined the facilities of A. L. Scovill & Co.'s laboratory, and found them sufficient and adequate to the demand of their business, being arranged upon the most approved scientific plan, which enables them to preserve all the various principles of the several agents entering into its combination as recommended by the highest Pharmaceutical authority in the United States and Europe."

NOTE.—With such testimony in its favor, coming, as it does, from high **medical authority,** and involving the certainty of its adoption and use by physicians in their regular practice, and in their **COLLEGES** and **HOSPITALS,** it may well be asked, why should not *every man, woman, and child* use it who has *any disease* of the *system,* whether it be in the form of *pimples* on the face, or the worst forms of **SCROFULA** or **SYPHILIS,** or any other form caused by an *impure state of the Blood or deranged state of the Liver,* when, for a comparatively small expense, **SCOVILL'S COMPOUND EXTRACT OF SARSAPARILLA AND STILLINGIA,** or **BLOOD AND LIVER SYRUP** can be procured?

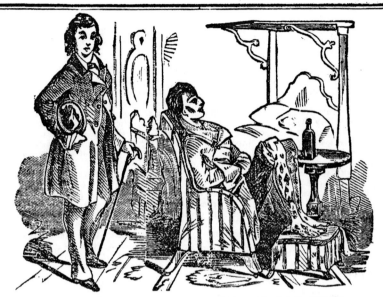

STILL ANOTHER TRULY REMARKABLE CURE

OF A

SCROFULOUS WHITE SWELLING!

The case was one so low that he could not turn in bed. The physicians pronounced him incurable. The statement was made to Dr. NEWTON, who happened to be at Dr. SCOVILL'S Office when Mr. James Whitaker related the whole case, which is as follows:

CINCINNATI, MARCH 29, 1860.

In June, 1858, he was attacked while at work in the field, complained of being tired, and of a heaviness; he then became confined to his bed until next winter.

Upon the hip there was a swelling, resembling a boil; this lasted for a few days without suppurating. Then the inflammation on the hip subsided, and it began to appear on the ankle; this became much swollen, and was attended with violent pain, which lasted about ten days, at which time suppuration was established, and it was lanced by his physician. After this, there was extensive discharge of matter from **twelve fistulous openings,** from the foot to the knee, so much so, that by inserting the pipe of the syringe, when filled with water, at the lower orifice, the water flowed freely from every opening, showing a complete communication. So extensive was this, that the flesh or muscles appeared to be separated from the bone. At this date the physician pronounced him incurable, unless **he** would consent to have his leg amputated, and this he stated to the boy and his friends.

Even while the doctor advised amputation, he acknowledged that there was but little hope even from that! The doctor stated to his neighbors that the boy could not live a month without it. My son objected to any operation, and there being no other hope, he began the use of **Scovill's Blood and Liver Syrup** in the last week in December, 1858. At that time he was confined to his bed, not able to stand on his feet, or even to turn himself over; loss of appetite, restless at night, with a free and extensive ulceration of the bone; over one hundred pieces have sloughed off, with all the attendant difficulties upon such a condition.

His condition is as follows: He is able to go any where he pleases, has regained his usual strength, his appetite is good, the suppuration of the leg is arrested, except in three small places, attended with but little discharge, only enough to stain the dressing in the twenty-four hours.

I now regard my son as well. This is one of the most desperate cases of scrofulous disease of the bone ever cured! One very remarkable feature of this case is, that the leg has regained its natural size and length, and there is not the least deformity of the limb. JAMES H. WHITAKER.

NOTE.—SCOVILL'S BLOOD AND LIVER SYRUP was the only medicine used.

Messrs. A. L. SCOVILL & Co.   CINCINNATI, JULY 11, 1861.

Gentlemen: Some two years ago my entire system became entirely **prostrated,** attended with disease of the **Liver, Spine** and **Kidneys.** The spine and kidneys caused me to **lose the use of my limbs, and I became bed-ridden** for more than a year. In this condition my **liver** and **digestive organs** became most **seriously diseased!** My Doctor, with two other Physicians, after holding consultation, **GAVE ME UP TO DIE, and advised me to prepare my business for death!** In this prostrated condition, confined to my bed, *suffering with pain more than of a thousand deaths, and, comparatively, more dead than alive, and, for months, not expecting to live,* was I, when I obtained a bottle of your BLOOD AND LIVER SYRUP, which was in February last, and from the very first I commenced gaining rapidly. The diseases in my **kidneys, liver, spine,** and **stomach, are ALL GETTING BETTER,** and I have only used seven bottles of your BLOOD AND LIVER SYRUP, at the same time bathing over my spine and kidneys with your DR. BAKER'S PAIN PANACEA. I am now able to go about as usual, and **feel so much better that I consider myself well.**

When I consider **how low** I have been, and the length of time that I was confined to bed helpless as a child, and the cure effected by your BLOOD AND LIVER SYRUP, **I FEEL THAT THE WORLD SHOULD KNOW IT!** and I believe that others who are afflicted will find **great benefit by its use.**

My residence is No. 98 East Third Street.

                                        Most truly yours,
                                                GEO. P. WARNER.

DR. SCOVILL.   PARKERSBURG, VA., JUNE 11, 1861.

Dear Sir: I have been **much afflicted with the SCROFULA** for some three years, and have tried almost *every preparation presented to afflicted mortality,* and, indeed, **have consulted the very BEST MEDICAL MEN OF THE AGE,** and received no benefit, until I accidentally tried your BLOOD AND LIVER SYRUP, **which indeed has acted like a charm!**

For some two years my neck and breast was covered with sores and ulcers. My physical strength was so prostrated that I could hardly **raise myself up in bed; my limbs were very sore and painful, and indeed my mind was so seriously affected that my most intimate friends thought that I had, to a great extent, lost the use of my reasoning faculty!** My stomach was also so affected that it appeared that ulcers had formed, which caused me to vomit from one to three times a day for some two years, but before **I had taken one bottle of your** BLOOD AND LIVER SYRUP, **the tone of my stomach was restored!** And now, with prudence, I can eat almost anything. **The ulcers and sores on my neck are almost entirely healed up. The soreness of my limbs has entirely left me,** and I flatter myself that I shall soon again be a sound man.

Send me two gallons of your BLOOD AND LIVER SYRUP, **and say to the world that your medicine can and will cure Dyspepsia and Scrofula!**

        Believe me, dear sir, your ob'd't serv't,   J. W. HORNER.

P. S.—The two gallons I wish for a friend, who is in a worse condition than I was, if possible. Physicians have given him up, and your Blood and Liver Syrup is the only thing which will cure him.   J. W. H.

N. B.—Mr Horner is an eminent lawyer, and ex-member of the Legislature of Virginia, and his statements can be relied upon as correct in every particular.

☞ How often people seem to live as though their happiness depended upon the amount of money which they are laboring to gain. Can we enjoy money without health?

In this country there are but few people, who use the proper means, that can not supply all their necessary wants, yet paying but little attention to diseases, which are gradually destroying the system. If the Liver and the secretions have been clogged, or the blood has accumulated humors, which engender Scrofula, cutaneous eruption, or liver complaint, by using SCOVILL'S BLOOD AND LIVER SYRUP the system can be restored to health, and without health money will be of little value.—*Statesman, Columbus, Ohio.*

COOPER'S PLAINS, STEUBEN Co., N. Y., March 1, 1860.
It is with pleasure that I write you in regard to Scovill's Blood and Liver Syrup. I think it one of the best purifiers of the day. It has met with perfect success in every case where I have used it. My first case was that of a young child, about eighteen months old, troubled with Erysipelas and Scrofula very badly. By the use of the Blood and Liver Syrup it has entirely recovered. The other case was a lady who had been afflicted with Scrofula for the last twenty-five years. She had tried the prescriptions of the most skillful physicians in this part of the country with no beneficial effect. She commenced using the Blood and Liver Syrup in November, and at that time was in the most deplorable condition—having been unable to do any work for the past twenty years. She is now entirely well, and able to attend to her work. S. W. EVERETT, M. D.

We have been particular in giving a few of the many cases that have come under our observation, and also a few extracts of the many letters that have been received respecting this compound, that it might be seen by the readers of this Journal that other physicians have used it with as much success as we have.

Although we recommend this preparation as a medicine for the people, still there are cases so complicated that other remedies may be necessary to be used in connection with this. In such cases, the patient should consult his physician, or correspond with the proprietors of this medicine. R. S. NEWTON, M. D., EDITOR.

—————

We have received the following certificate from DR. SAMUEL SILSBEE, who devotes especial attention to the treatment of Scrofula, Syphilitic Skin Diseases, and all chronic diseases arising from an impure state of the blood:
"I have carefully examined your *formula* for SYRUP OF SARSAPARILLA AND STILLINGIA, and have used it in my practice, and found it the MOST VALUABLE ALTERATIVE in *Scrofula and Syphilitic Diseases* that I have ever used. I have no hesitation in recommending it to PHYSICIANS and others."
CINCINNATI, Sept. 1, 1858. SAMUEL SILSBEE, M. D.
Office South side Sixth Street, between Main and Walnut.

REMARKABLE CURE OF ERYSIPELAS.
Below read the statement of Mr. BENJAMIN HOPKINS, a merchant of Cincinnati, No. 139, Main Street:
MESSRS. A. L. SCOVILL & Co.
Gentlemen:—Knowing that many are suffering, as I have been, from that TROUBLESOME DISEASE, ERYSIPELAS, who would be glad to find a *sure remedy*, I feel it my duty to make the following statement:
I have long been afflicted with ERYSIPELAS, and have tried various remedies, *without effecting a cure.* I have used only *two bottles* of your COMPOUND EXTRACT of SARSAPARILLA and STILLINGIA or BLOOD SYRUP, which has *completely cured me.* At the same time I was afflicted with the DYSPEPSIA, *which it has also cured.*
CINCINNATI, O., September 19, 1858. BENJAMIN E. HOPKINS.

—————

Certificate from Dr. James S. Ewan, of Hardiugburg, Indiana, well known in his vicinity.
HARDINGBURG, September 9, 1858.
MESSRS. A. L. SCOVILL & Co.
Gents:—This is to certify that I have been using *Scovill's Sarsaparilla and Stillingia* in my practice, and find that in every case where I have used it, it has worked like a charm, and would recommend it to all afflicted with Chronic or Consumptive diseases. JAMES S. EWAN, M. D.

—————

WAREHAM, MASS., January 27, 1860.
MESSRS. A. L. SCOVILL & Co.
I have never, in my life, taken much medicine. I saw the circular recommending your Blood and Liver Syrup, and I made up my mind that it would suit my case. About six years ago I had a prickly feeling in my legs, and if I remained still for ten minutes my legs became numb and palsied. It kept me in a complete nervous uneasiness, and at night my blood would become stagnated, which affected my head and back. I would turn over and over at least twenty times during the night. Twelve months since, while I was actively employed, I had so severe an attack that I have not been able to exercise since without producing much pain. I commenced taking your Blood and Liver Syrup, and have taken a few bottles; and believe me, Mr. Scovill, I am entirely well, and feel better than at any time for the last fifteen years. A. C. FEARING.

4

SCROFULA CURED!

Messrs. A. L. Scovill & Co.:   Cincinnati, April 12, 1859.

Gents: From a sense of duty, I give you a statement of a cure of my son by the use of your BLOOD and LIVER SYRUP. He was taken about three years ago with the SCROFULA; sores made their appearance upon the side of his neck, under the skin, which was hard and red, (or inflamed.) We called upon one of our first physicians of this city, who treated him, but the sores, under his treatment, became ULCERS, and broke and discharged.

The physician did all he could, but the sufferer continued to get weak and poor and had but little appetite. I called on another, in consultation, but without any better success. I had nearly given up all hopes of HIS GETTING WELL.

Some three months ago, some one of my neighbors was telling of the cures made by your BLOOD and LIVER SYRUP. I got a bottle, and found that his appetite began to be much better, also his color, and by the use of ten bottles *he has been cured !*
JAMES REILY,
Lower Market, between Main and Sycamore.

Mr. JAMES D. LEHMER, one of our oldest wholesale merchants, doing business on Columbia street, one door west of Vine street, states that HIS SON had been SCROFULOUS for many years, and sores came upon his neck. He had the best of medical treatment, but without success in curing him. He then got SCOVILL'S BL__D and LIVER SYRUP, and the result is, he is effectually cured. He considers the operation of this medicine *truly remarkable on his son.*

THE BLOOD AND LIVER SYRUP

NOT ONLY CLEANSES THE SYSTEM, BUT REMOVES UNNATURAL TUMORS, SUCH AS GOITRE OR SWELLED NECK, Etc.

GOITRE OR SWELLED NECK CURED.

Cincinnati, March 12, 1859.

Messrs. A. L. Scovill & Co.:

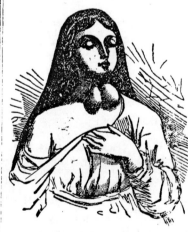

Dear Sirs: My daughter had a LARGE SWELLING, or GOITRE, coming on her neck during the last four years.

Our PHYSICIAN used his uttermost skill in trying to cure her, BUT FAILED.

Your BLOOD and LIVER SYRUP was highly recommended to me. I made up my mind to give it a trial. I bought a bottle, and she commenced to use it. After this I could see THAT THE DISEASE was MUCH ABATED. I then got more, and used externally the ointment, as directed. After taking ten or twelve bottles she was entirely cured.   JAMES BATES,
Fifth St., between Plum and Western Row.

Note.—The above certificate shows how admirably this medicine acts on the *system.* Its action is through the secretion of the absorbent vessels, and consists in receiving or taking up certain substances, known as virus, or poisonous principles, and removing them from the diseased parts, through the secretions and exhalant arteries, until they are carried from the system.

We also refer to A. B. EATON, Esq., of this city, a merchant largely known, and a DEACON in the REVEREND MR. STORRS' CONGREGATIONAL CHURCH, respecting the *cure of his daughter* of GOITRE or SWELLED NECK, by the use of the BLOOD and LIVER SYRUP.

Mr. A. B. EATON'S residence is on Smith, three doors below Longworth street, Cincinnati.

SCROFULOUS SORE EYES CURED!

The Testimony of a well-known Merchant of Kentucky.

HAGENSVILLE, Bracken county, Kentucky, March 3, 1859.
MESSRS. A. L. SCOVILL & Co.:

Dear Sirs: My daughter has been afflicted with SCROFULOUS SORE EYES and FACE; also other sores on different parts of her BODY. I have been using your BLOOD and LIVER SYRUP, and it has PURIFIED HER BLOOD, and made an entire cure of her. I have no hesitancy in recommending this medicine in all cases of Scrofula, or any *diseases* of the *Blood.*

I give you this statement, believing that *so valuable a medicine* ought to be made known to the PUBLIC.   M. HAGEN.

Two Children Cured of Scrofula.

MESSRS. A. L. SCOVILL & Co.:   CINCINNATI, March 4, 1859.

Dear Sirs: This is to certify that my two children have been afflicted with SCROFULOUS ULCERS. I tried your BLOOD and LIVER SYRUP, which CURED *them in a remarkably* SHORT TIME. And my wife has been using it for the *Tetter* and *Rheumatism,* and is now well. If any one wants a medicine for PURIFYING the BLOOD, they will find the above named among the BEST NOW IN USE.
                     JAMES G. MISENER,

Formerly of the firm of TRAINER & MISENER, two doors below the Gibson House.

Scrofulous Sore Neck Cured.

MESSRS. A. L. SCOVILL & Co.:   CINCINNATI, January 30, 1858.

Gents: Your medicine has made a wonderful cure of my son. He was taken with a Scrofulous sore on the glands of the neck. We tried different remedies, and yet it seemed to get worse. I tried your BLOOD SYRUP, by taking it three times a day, and also applying the *Iodide of Potassium Ointment,* externally to the parts. By the use of six bottles of your BLOOD SYRUP, he was cured. I write you this statement that others may know of your valuable medicine.   Yours,
                     JAMES BENNETT,
                     Lower Market, between Broadway and Sycamore.

Inflammatory Rheumatism Cured.

MESSRS. A. L. SCOVILL & Co.:   CINCINNATI, July 10, 1857.

Gentlemen: This is to certify that I was last winter afflicted with Inflammatory Rheumatism for eight weeks. I tried almost everything that was recommended to me, but found no relief. I was confined to bed, and my legs were very much swollen, attended with excruciating pain. I tried your BLOOD SYRUP, and used the *Stimulating Liniment* as directed; and by the use of three bottles of your BLOOD SYRUP was perfectly cured. I enjoy better health than ever.
                     PETER KENNEDY,
                     Fifth Street, between Main and Walnut.

A Physician's Testimony.

MESSRS. A. L. SCOVILL & Co.:   WELLSBURG, Virginia, January 13, 1859.

Gentlemen: I have used all of your *Sarsaparilla* and *Stillingia,* or BLOOD and LIVER SYRUP, you sent me, in my practice, and find that it *gives better satisfaction for those diseases for which it is recommended than any other medicine we ever sold.* Please to ship me another lot *immediately.*   G. W. CALDWELL, M. D.

DR. WM. HALL'S

BALSAM FOR THE LUNGS,

FOR THE CURE OF

Consumption, Decline, Asthma, Bronchitis, Wasting of Flesh, Night-Sweats, Spitting of Blood, Hooping Cough, Difficulty of Breathing, Colds, Cough, Influenza, Phthisic, Pain in the Side, and all Diseases of the Lungs.

10,000 DOLLARS REWARD

IS OFFERED FOR A BETTER RECIPE.

IT CONTAINS NO OPIUM, CALOMEL, OR MINERAL POISON!

AND IS SAFE FOR THE MOST DELICATE CHILD!

IT is estimated that 150,000 persons die annually in the United States, with consumption, and Professor Eberly says, that a vast number of these could be saved by the timely use of some proper remedy.

DR. HALL'S BALSAM strikes at the root of the disease at once, and such is its speedy effect, that any one using it freely, according to directions, for twenty-four or forty-eight hours, and not entirely satisfied with its merits may return it and receive back his money. The most distressing cough is frequently relieved by a single dose, and broken up in a few hours' time. The afflicted do not have to take bottle after bottle before they find whether this remedy will afford relief or not.

Call on the agent and get a pamphlet gratis. The treatise on consumption alone is worth the price for the medicine. You will find certificates of physicians in Cincinnati, and of others whose cures have been effected here at home, where they can be found.

The public have been imposed upon by remedies recommended by certificates which have always originated from some unknown source. We believe that a medicine possessing real merits will effect cures wherever it is used, at home as well as abroad. This is no paregoric preparation, but one which, if used in season, will save the lives of thousands; and persons may make this bargain with agents from whom they purchase; that, in every case where it is used freely, according to directions, and entire satisfaction is not given in twenty-four or forty-eight hours, they can return the medicine, and their money will be cheerfully refunded.

It has effected cures in numerous cases, where the most skillful physicians in this country and in Europe have been employed, and have exercised their skill in vain. Cases which they pronounced incurable, and surrendered as hopeless beyond a doubt, leaving the patients without a single ray to enliven them in their gloom, have been cured by DR. HALL'S BALSAM, and the "victims of consumption" are now vigorous and strong as the most robust among us. And these cases are not isolated ones; they are numerous, and can be pointed out in every community, where this most unrivaled remedy has been tested.

Be slow, then, to believe the oft-repeated story about the lungs being gone; or rather let no such apprehension induce you to give up. Act upon the principle that while there is life there is hope. You can never be so low that you may not trust, humanly speaking, in HALL'S BALSAM. More than one, nay hundreds, has it brought almost from death to life, when all else had failed. Give, then, this powerful but harmless remedy a trial.

We have certificates of its cures from many of our most respectable citizens—men and women who live and have been cured among us. For particulars, we refer those living out of the city to our agents. Against such preparations as never effect cures where they had their origin, we would caution you. Unknown persons and places, and fictitious cases, are made subservient to the spread and use of remedies of this doubtful character.

Accompanying each bottle of DR. HALL'S BALSAM instruction, in pamphlet form, on consumption, with directions for using, modes, treatments, etc., for which we bespeak your perusal.

CONSUMPTION
A
CURABLE DISEASE!

WE are aware that a contrary opinion has been long and generally entertained. The teaching of the medical schools, from time immemorial, has been, that *Pulmonary Consumption* is *incurable.* The learned Professor has gravely declared this as the truth, and the youthful disciple has received it, without even *daring* to question its correctness.

Hence, also, the general impression among the community, that Consumption is incurable. No sooner does the unfortunate patient begin to perceive, in his *dry hacking cough, pains in the side and breast, spitting of blood, night-sweats,* etc., the unmistakable signs of diseased lungs, than he concludes, forthwith, that he has *Consumption;* and because he has it, immediately abandons himself to despair, without even thinking to inquire whether a beneficent Creator has not mercifully vouchsafed to his suffering children a remedy for *this,* as well as every other ill which afflicts diseased humanity.

But the motto of the present age is ONWARD! Old stereotyped opinions, which have nothing but their *antiquity* to recommend them, are fast giving way, as their absurdities are proved by the searching investigations of science. The Steam Car, the Railroad, the Magnetic Telegraph, are revolutionizing the earth. And while the human mind has been busy in every department of the Physical Sciences, producing results which have *astonished the world,* think you that Medicine is the only science which has stood still? Are *we* now no wiser than were our *fathers?* Has the accumulated research of the nineteenth century thrown no light upon the *Practice of Medicine?*

We do not say that *every single case* of Consumption (at an *advanced stage,* and where the patient has a scrofulous constitution) *can be cured;* but *we* DO SAY, that where the general health of the system is not fatally disordered, and where there is sufficient vital energy left, *Consumption* is *as curable as any other disease!* Patients occasionally die of *Bilious Fever,* yet we account it a *curable disease,* because the *majority,* if treated rightly, *recover.* So we say of *Consumption.* By the timely administration of this medicine, every *recent* case can be *speedily* and *thoroughly cured;* and through all the various stages of the complaint, from a simple Cough, or a *neglected Cold,* down to the most hopeless case of confirmed, tuberculous Consumption.

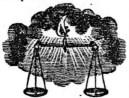

READER! have you a cough, which you are neglecting, under the idea that it is only a common cold, and that it will soon "wear itself out?" Let a friend tell you, in all kindness, what will soon be the probable result. In a short time, if you continue to neglect yourself, you will begin to feel a sense of tightness and oppression across the chest, accompanied with frequent sharp darting pains. Then, a dry, hacking cough will set in, and when you raise anything, it will be a thick and yellowish, or white frothy matter, streaked, perhaps, with blood. If you still take no medicine, these unpleasant symptoms will increase, and you will soon have hectic fever, cold chills, night-sweats, copious expectoration, and then great prostration. If you still neglect yourself, a few weeks or months will see you consigned to the grave, leaving your friends to mourn how rapidly Consumption did its work, and hurried you away. Friend! have you no cause to be alarmed? In the above sketch you may see as in a glass, how every case of Consumption progresses, with more or less rapidity, to a fatal termination. Of all the thousands and millions whom this great destroyer has gathered to the tomb, every single case began with a cold! If this had been attended to, all might have been well; but, being neglected, under the fatal delusion that it would "wear itself off," it transferred its deadly action to the substance of the lungs, exciting there the formation of tubercles. Another and another cold added fuel to the flame, until these tubercles began to soften and suppurate, leaving, by their ulceration, great cavities in the lungs. At this crisis the disease is very difficult of cure, and oftentimes sets at defiance all human means.

In the latter, or worst stage, this medicine will oftentimes arrest the disease, or check its progress, and will always make the patient more comfortable, and prolong his life, and it is therefore worthy of a trial; but in its incipient or forming periods, Consumption is as curable as any other disease, and **Dr. HALL'S Balsam for the Lungs,** if taken at this time, will cure it as surely as it is taken!

THE LUNGS

ARE THE

GREAT LABORATORY OF THE SYSTEM.

THE cause of death, by Consumption, is the collection and continuation of numerous small sores in the lungs (lights) and pulmonary vessels, (veins, or blood, or air vessels which run through the lungs.) These sores (called tubercles) are swellings of a dull yellowish or whitish appearance, rather hard at first, but after a while they become soft and produce a running ulcer, the matter from which excites coughing and is raised in a yellowish ropy matter-like expectoration. In some cases the ulcers destroy entirely one part of the lungs, and still the patient can live, though rarely, for some time, with only the use of half the lungs. These sores commence in small hard kernels, from the size of a pea to a minute speck, called *semi-transparent granulations*.

The kernels form the first stage, and as they are frequently very thick, a number sometimes unite as they enlarge, and form one extensive corroding sore. As the sores enlarge, they embrace some of the blood-vessels, which run through the lungs in all directions, and whenever these are destroyed or eaten off, there is *bleeding at the lungs*.

When a large vein happens to burst by being rotted away by the sore, death frequently happens very soon. These kernels always appear first in the upper part of the lungs, and when these get to be sores, other kernels or white hard specks form lower down. These bodies present, in the early stage, a gray semi-transparent substance, which gradually becomes yellow, opaque, and dense; it afterward softens and gradually becomes converted into a fluid, like thick cream or pus, which, being expelled through the air vessels by coughing, leaves cavities in the lungs, which may be termed ulcers. Dr. C. Draper says: "By neglecting those salutary precautions which common sense dictates, many, very many, fall victims to their imprudence. We have seen the young bride, blooming, as it were, as the bird of paradise, and the fair flower of hope, the pride of her father, and the joy of her mother; her cheek flushed with anticipations, and her eye beaming with the soft expressions of love; the gay dreams of life dancing on her fancy, with the rich and variegated tints of the rainbow's promise; we have seen all this changed, ay, the wedding garment changed for a shroud, and the bridal-chamber for the sepulcher of the dead—and all this from *neglecting a common cold.*"

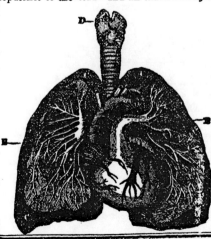

HEALTHY LUNGS.

THIS cut represents the lungs in a healthy state. **B B**, the lung or air cells. **C C**, the covering of the lungs.

It is estimated that the whole number of these air cells in the lungs, is about six hundred millions; and if these air cells were cut open, they would cover the space of twenty thousand square inches.

DR. BAKER'S
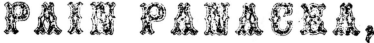
PAIN PANACEA,

FOR THE CURE OF PAIN,

BOTH EXTERNALLY AND INTERNALLY.

THE GREATEST PAIN-CURING REMEDY
YET DISCOVERED!!

Pain cannot long Exist where this Remedy is Faithfully Used.

☞GIVE IT ONE FAIR TRIAL,☜

And if you do not find it to be all it is recommended, go back to the Agent and get

DOUBLE THE AMOUNT OF MONEY REFUNDED!

This offer is made knowing that what this medicine has done in thousands of cases, it will do again.

FOR PAIN
IN THE STOMACH, BACK AND BOWELS,

Burns, Bruises, Cuts and Swellings, Colic, Diarrhea, and Rheumatism, Headache, Toothache, and Earache,

IT CURES ALMOST INSTANTANEOUSLY!

CHRONIC DISEASES,
SUCH AS

Dyspepsia, Weak Breast, Liver Complaint, General Debility, Fever and Ague, Canker or Sore Mouth, Putrid Sore Throat, Weak Eyes, Spine and Kidney Disease, Old Sores, Coughs and Colds.

In the above-named Diseases it needs only to be faithfully used, and

A CURE IS CERTAIN!!

MONEY REFUNDED!

IMPORTANT TO AGENTS.—Agents will find it greatly to their interest, and are at full liberty, on first introducing DR. BAKER'S PAIN PANACEA, to give back the money freely, if those who purchase it are not fully satisfied ; and may use it in their own FAMILIES, or give a few bottles to their friends, that they may test its GREAT MERITS over all other remedies ; and, when once introduced, they will find that they can sell large quantities of it. All Agents write that, when once introduced, their sales are large. Families will keep it in their houses, and will not be without it.

DIRECTIONS
Are fully given and particularly adapted to the different diseases for which the Panacea is recommended

CPSIA information can be obtained
at www.ICGtesting.com
Printed in the USA
LVOW10s1526260318
571183LV00056B/1746/P

9 780260 195210